The Pythagorean diet, of vegetables only, conducive to the preservation of health, and the cure of diseases. A discourse delivered at Florence, in the month of August, 1743, by Antonio Cocchi, ... Translated from the Italian.

Antonio Cocchi

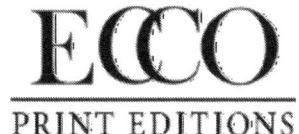

The Pythagorean diet, of vegetables only, conducive to the preservation of health, and the cure of diseases. A discourse delivered at Florence, in the month of August, 1743, by Antonio Cocchi, ... Translated from the Italian.
Cocchi, Antonio
ESTCID: T143720
Reproduction from British Library

London : printed for R. Dodsley; and sold by M. Cooper, 1745.
[4],91,[1]p. ; 8°

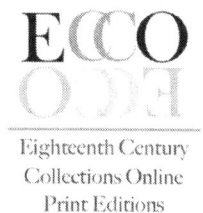

Eighteenth Century
Collections Online
Print Editions

Gale ECCO Print Editions

Relive history with *Eighteenth Century Collections Online*, now available in print for the independent historian and collector. This series includes the most significant English-language and foreign-language works printed in Great Britain during the eighteenth century, and is organized in seven different subject areas including literature and language; medicine, science, and technology; and religion and philosophy. The collection also includes thousands of important works from the Americas.

The eighteenth century has been called "The Age of Enlightenment." It was a period of rapid advance in print culture and publishing, in world exploration, and in the rapid growth of science and technology – all of which had a profound impact on the political and cultural landscape. At the end of the century the American Revolution, French Revolution and Industrial Revolution, perhaps three of the most significant events in modern history, set in motion developments that eventually dominated world political, economic, and social life.

In a groundbreaking effort, Gale initiated a revolution of its own: digitization of epic proportions to preserve these invaluable works in the largest online archive of its kind. Contributions from major world libraries constitute over 175,000 original printed works. Scanned images of the actual pages, rather than transcriptions, recreate the works ***as they first appeared.***

Now for the first time, these high-quality digital scans of original works are available via print-on-demand, making them readily accessible to libraries, students, independent scholars, and readers of all ages.

For our initial release we have created seven robust collections to form one the world's most comprehensive catalogs of 18th century works.

Initial Gale ECCO Print Editions collections include:

> ***History and Geography***
> Rich in titles on English life and social history, this collection spans the world as it was known to eighteenth-century historians and explorers. Titles include a wealth of travel accounts and diaries, histories of nations from throughout the world, and maps and charts of a world that was still being discovered. Students of the War of American Independence will find fascinating accounts from the British side of conflict.

Social Science
Delve into what it was like to live during the eighteenth century by reading the first-hand accounts of everyday people, including city dwellers and farmers, businessmen and bankers, artisans and merchants, artists and their patrons, politicians and their constituents. Original texts make the American, French, and Industrial revolutions vividly contemporary.

Medicine, Science and Technology
Medical theory and practice of the 1700s developed rapidly, as is evidenced by the extensive collection, which includes descriptions of diseases, their conditions, and treatments. Books on science and technology, agriculture, military technology, natural philosophy, even cookbooks, are all contained here.

Literature and Language
Western literary study flows out of eighteenth-century works by Alexander Pope, Daniel Defoe, Henry Fielding, Frances Burney, Denis Diderot, Johann Gottfried Herder, Johann Wolfgang von Goethe, and others. Experience the birth of the modern novel, or compare the development of language using dictionaries and grammar discourses.

Religion and Philosophy
The Age of Enlightenment profoundly enriched religious and philosophical understanding and continues to influence present-day thinking. Works collected here include masterpieces by David Hume, Immanuel Kant, and Jean-Jacques Rousseau, as well as religious sermons and moral debates on the issues of the day, such as the slave trade. The Age of Reason saw conflict between Protestantism and Catholicism transformed into one between faith and logic -- a debate that continues in the twenty-first century.

Law and Reference
This collection reveals the history of English common law and Empire law in a vastly changing world of British expansion. Dominating the legal field is the *Commentaries of the Law of England* by Sir William Blackstone, which first appeared in 1765. Reference works such as almanacs and catalogues continue to educate us by revealing the day-to-day workings of society.

Fine Arts
The eighteenth-century fascination with Greek and Roman antiquity followed the systematic excavation of the ruins at Pompeii and Herculaneum in southern Italy; and after 1750 a neoclassical style dominated all artistic fields. The titles here trace developments in mostly English-language works on painting, sculpture, architecture, music, theater, and other disciplines. Instructional works on musical instruments, catalogs of art objects, comic operas, and more are also included.

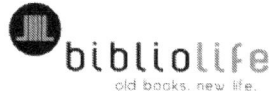

The BiblioLife Network

This project was made possible in part by the BiblioLife Network (BLN), a project aimed at addressing some of the huge challenges facing book preservationists around the world. The BLN includes libraries, library networks, archives, subject matter experts, online communities and library service providers. We believe every book ever published should be available as a high-quality print reproduction; printed on-demand anywhere in the world. This insures the ongoing accessibility of the content and helps generate sustainable revenue for the libraries and organizations that work to preserve these important materials.

The following book is in the "public domain" and represents an authentic reproduction of the text as printed by the original publisher. While we have attempted to accurately maintain the integrity of the original work, there are sometimes problems with the original work or the micro-film from which the books were digitized. This can result in minor errors in reproduction. Possible imperfections include missing and blurred pages, poor pictures, markings and other reproduction issues beyond our control. Because this work is culturally important, we have made it available as part of our commitment to protecting, preserving, and promoting the world's literature.

GUIDE TO FOLD-OUTS MAPS and OVERSIZED IMAGES

The book you are reading was digitized from microfilm captured over the past thirty to forty years. Years after the creation of the original microfilm, the book was converted to digital files and made available in an online database.

In an online database, page images do not need to conform to the size restrictions found in a printed book. When converting these images back into a printed bound book, the page sizes are standardized in ways that maintain the detail of the original. For large images, such as fold-out maps, the original page image is split into two or more pages

Guidelines used to determine how to split the page image follows:

• Some images are split vertically; large images require vertical and horizontal splits.
• For horizontal splits, the content is split left to right.
• For vertical splits, the content is split from top to bottom.
• For both vertical and horizontal splits, the image is processed from top left to bottom right.

THE
Pythagorean DIET,
OF
VEGETABLES
ONLY,

Conducive to the PRESERVATION
of HEALTH,

And the *CURE* of *DISEASES*.

A Discourse delivered at *Florence*, in the
Month of *August*, 1743,

By *ANTONIO COCCHI*, of *Mugello*.

Translated from the ITALIAN.

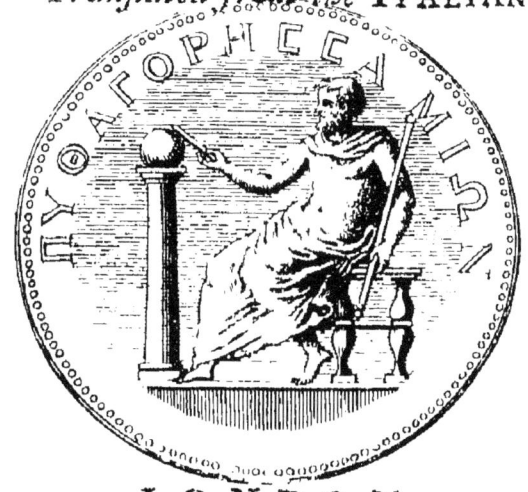

LONDON:
Printed for R. Dodsley, in *Pall Mall*; and
sold by M. Cooper, at the *Globe* in *Pater-
noster Row*. M,DCC,XLV.

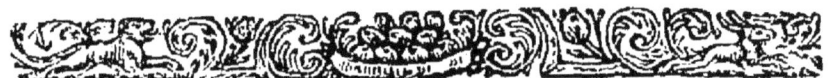

THE following Discourse having been received in Italy with a great deal of Approbation, 'tis presumed the English Reader will be pleased to meet with it in his own Language. The Author was some Years ago in England, is now Keeper of the Great Duke of Tuscany's Musæum, a Fellow of our Royal Society, as well as of the College of Physicians in Florence, and will be found to speak of the English Nation in the highest Terms of Respect.

A DISCOURSE ON THE DIET OF THE *PYTHAGOREANS.*

PYTHAGORAS was certainly one of the greatest Geniuses that ever Human Nature produc'd. He liv'd about 500 Years before the Birth of *Christ*, near which Time History began to be written with Truth and Clearness;

whereas, in the Ages preceding, it had most commonly been deliver'd in a poetical, fabulous, and obscure manner.

The Writings of the Authors cotemporary with him, are now in a manner all lost, nor have we any Account of them, but at second hand, from such as liv'd long after. Experience daily teaches us, that the greatest Part of Mankind are inclin'd, by a certain natural mean Envy, to detract from the Praise of others, and especially of those who are the most illustrious, by malicious or false Aspersions, whilst many others are induc'd, through Stupidity and Ignorance, to imagine and believe such Aspersions true, altho' they are without Foundation, and absurd. It is also observable, that obscure and allegorical Expressions are always liable to be interpreted according to the literal Meaning of the Words, and in a manner very different from the Intention of the Author.

Hence it is, that in the Course of so many Ages, the History of *Pythagoras* is

found

found perplex'd with such Numbers of strange and incredible Circumstances, and that the Doctrines of his School, which were deliver'd in a figurative manner of Expression, have been so alter'd, that it is no wonder, if, in the Books we read of him, he appears sometimes as (1) a Worker of Miracles by virtue of his Goodness, at other times as a ridiculous (2) Wizard and Impostor, and that many who think of him the most favourably, consider him no otherwise than as a fantastical and obscure Philosopher.

But if we seek industriously at the Fountain-Head, for whatever Information concerning him is scatter'd amongst many Writers, and judge thereof according to the Rules of true Criticism, excluding every thing that has a direct Repugnancy to the Nature of the Case, we shall easily be perswaded, that he came up very near to

---

(1) Jamblici Vitâ de Pythag. καὶ ταῦτα μὲν ἐςι τεκμήρια τῆς εὐσεβείας αὐτῦ.

(2) *Laertius*, and the Authors cited in the Notes of the *Menagiana*.

to the Perfection of that Character which is so rarely to be met with, and which results from an Union of the most generous and beneficent Qualities of the Heart, in the most extensive and well-grounded Knowledge and Understanding.

His Doctrine consisted, in possessing, in a high degree, those three Parts whereinto all Human Wisdom may readily be divided, as he first of all divided it, *viz*. Erudition, or the Art of Thinking and Speaking, Philosophy, or the Knowledge of the Nature of Things, and Civil Prudence, or the Understanding of Government, and the Laws and Duties which result from (1) Society. And if he was excellent in critical and moral Knowledge, so much the more shall we find him wonderful in the Knowledge of Nature, as that sort of Knowledge exceeds the other two in Difficulty and Extensiveness.

Tho' none, it seems, of the entire and authentic Works of *Pythagoras* have been read,

---

(3) *Laertius*, lib viii sect 6

read, nevertheless in the Writings of those learned Men, whom we call the Antients, there remain such Vestiges of his Philosophy, as taught by his Scholars, and the Fame is so constant of his Authority for certain particular Opinions that we may without Rashness, even at this Day, form a Judgment of his Worth.

He was an excellent Mathematician; and improv'd Geometry very much by his Inventions on the Elements laid down by the *Egyptians*, and made Use of Arithmetic as a universal and analytical way of calculating. He was a great Philosopher and Astronomer, and also understood Natural History and Physic, which is no other than the Result of various learned Observations, join'd with common Prudence.

It is indeed true, that his Doctrines were, by him and his Followers, designedly concealed from the Knowledge of the common People, under the Veil of strange Expressions, understood only by his School, and that the Sense of his Doctrines be-

came

came obscure soon after, from there being only a verbal, not a written Explanation of them. If we could possibly know the Circumstances on which it is founded, we should understand much better the Connexion of this his Closeness with his Philosophy, which now seems to us extravagant and dangerous in its Nature. It may be, the Pleasure of doing good to others, or even the Love of Praise, which great Souls are generally the most desirous of, induc'd him not to suppress certain important Truths, however proper it might be to conceal them from the Multitude, which was thought antiently uncapable of being any otherwise instructed than through the Means of some Falshood, universally insinuated with a useful kind of Fallacy, and then spread Abroad, and supported more and more by all possible Machinery and Invention.

And because all Truths are connected one with another, and assist each other for the expelling and abolishing of Falshood, and that

that all sovereign Powers have, from the Nature of their Constitution, the free Distribution of coercive Force; on that Account, from that Time even to our own, not the *Pythagorean* only, but in a manner all Schools have found it absolutely necessary for their Preservation, to make Use of the famous Method of teaching two Doctrines, the one secret, and the other open; that which was taught at Home, clear and direct, and that which went Abroad, obscure, oblique, and involv'd in Symbols.

This Reflection should have render'd those more cautious, who (tho' otherwise ingenious) call the Doctrines of *Pythagoras* by the Names of Dreams and Follies; and as for those other silly Surmisers who have attributed Miracles and Inchantments to him, it would be a Folly to make any Mention of them in this distinguishing and penetrating Age. We may then discern through the Clouds wherewith this Philosopher endeavour'd to conceal his new and elevated Doctrines from the Eyes of the Vulgar, that he thought the Sun to be the Fire or lucid Center of our World, and the Earth a Planet, (1) and that Matter, being never deficient, compos'd other like Systems in the immense Ether. He supposes the Comets to be Planets, whose Returns have the longest Periods, (2) and concludes, that in the Motions of the Cælestial Bodies there is a determinate Harmony, (3) that is, a mutual relative Correspondence between their Sizes and Distances (4): He was the first that understood the Appearances of the Planet *Venus*, (5) that knew the *Earth* was of a nearly spherical Figure, and in an oblique Position, and that it was all over habitable, with an equal Distribution of Light and Darkness to all its Parts (6). He also was

---

(1) Aristot lib ii de Cælo & Plutarch in Num.
(2) Plutarch de Opinion Philosoph lib ii. 13 & Chalcid in Tim p 304
(3) Plutarch ibid lib iii 2
(4) Plin ii 21 & 22 Censorin 13
(5) Plin ibid & Laert vii 14
(6) Plutarch de Opinion Phil lib ii. 12 & Laert.

was the first, and the only one among all the Antients, who maintain'd that the Generation of Animals was constantly effected by the Means of Seeds from other Animals of the same Kind, and that such a Faculty could never be allow'd to any other sort of Matter; (1) which Sentiment being contrary to the System of the *Egyptians* from whom some would maintain that he borrow'd all his Opinions, it serves to prove, so much the more fully, the Power of his profound and sagacious Mind. And if more such sublime Ways of Thinking are to be found in the Philosophy of *Pythagoras*, (2) we should either forbear to attempt an Explanation of his other obscure

---

(1) Laert Sect 28

(2) These may be collected from the Authors before quoted, and from many other ancient Writers, without mentioning what the Commentators on *Laertius* have done, what *Scheffer* relates in his learned Book *de Natura & Constitutione Philosophiæ Pythagoricæ Ups 1664* And also that very wise Judgment concerning the Philosophy of *Pythagoras*, which we meet with in the Comment of *Chalcid in Tim. de Plat p* 395 *Pythagoras assistere veritati minus licet & contra opinionem pro iners opinantibus affectationibus non veretur*

scure Doctrines, or understand them in a Sense agreeable to these so strong and fertile Conceptions, or else suppose them not his, tho' imputed to him.

We should then have no other Idea of *Pythagoras* than that of his being a Mathematician, a Philosopher, and a Naturalist, as his Citizens of *Samos* have judiciously represented him upon their Money, (1) which we still meet with. He appears in the Figure of a venerable old Man, sitting, in the Habit of an Hero, with only a Mantle over him. In his left Hand he holds

---

(1) Of the Coins of the Isle of *Samos*, with the Figure of *Pythagoras*, one in Brass with the Head of *Etruscilla* is in the *Medicean* Collection of his Royal Highness the Great Duke of *Tuscany*, from which the Figure at the Beginning of this Treatise is copied, but enlarg'd to twice the Size. *Vaillant* has register'd six, besides one of *Nicæa* with the same Figure, and the Head of *Gallienus*, from the Antiquary *Camelli*, and another like one, if it be not the same, is mentioned in *Spanheim*, on the Authority of *Francesco-Gottifredi* de U & P N. Edit. 2 p 491. The same *Gottifredi* in a Manuscript Index to his Medals, made in 1652, thus describes it, *Figura Pythagoræ sedentis cum Globo* ΝΙΚΑΙΕΩΝ, ? mod. He that shall see such a Medal, and be well assured of the Truth of the Figures and the Reading, may then enquire into the Relation between the Citizens of *Nicæa* and *Pythagoras*.

holds a Sceptre, and in his Right a little Stick, wherewith he shews a Globe placed on a small Pillar, and seems as it were describing the Figure of the Earth, the Obliquity of the Ecliptic, or the Sphere and System of the World, and the Theory of the Stars, which he with so great Judgment had conceived.

And such, necessarily, must have been the Founder of the celebrated School of *Italy*, which, by an Application of Mathematics to Philosophy, has with Reason always maintained the highest Rank amongst all the several Sects of Philosophers, and has produced the best Mechanics, and the most penetrating Authors. As an Instance of which, we need only mention that Discourse of *Archimedes*, on Bodies floating in Water; and his other Works abundantly serve to confirm the same Truth: As also do the Remains of *Aristarchus*, with the Fragments or Sentiments of *Empedocles*, *Archytus*, and *Philolaus*, which are handed to us by Tradition,

dition, and those of many others whose precious Labours are now lost.

And as *Pythagoras* made a most shining Figure in the World as a Man of Learning and a Philosopher, from having join'd together so much and such (1) Knowledge, we cannot deny him the farther Praise of having been one of the most useful and most amiable Men that can be imagined in common Society. He was healthful, well made, and cleanly in his Person; had a Fortune of his own sufficient for one in a middling Condition, and was born of virtuous and honourable Parents. (2) He travelled through the most civilized and remote Nations, and consequently became well acquainted with the Virtues and Vices of Human Nature. He

was

---

(1) *Heraclitus*, a Philosopher, who lived in the Times nearest to that of *Pythagoras*, writes of him as *Laertius* attests, Lib viii 6 Πυταγόρης Μνησάρχου ἱστορίην ἤσκησεν ανθρώπων μάλιστα πάντων, that he was of all Men the most exercised in universal Knowledge.

(2) *Pausan* ii 13. All the rest of this Character is gather'd, and in a Manner translated from various Places in *Laertius*, *Porphyry*, and others of the Ancients

was the Father of a Family; moſt dear to his Relations; had a Wife and Children, and therefore thought himſelf obliged to be the more moderate and the more humane.

He was a remarkable Promoter of Benevolence and Friendſhip among his Acquaintance, ſweet and complaiſant in Converſation, never deriding nor ſcandalizing any Body, and extremely juſt in all his Actions, as may be learned by that celebrated Saying of his, "That a Man "ſhould always reſtrain himſelf from "breaking the Law, or taking Advantage "of any Prevarication therein." He was ſo generous, that he thought nothing he poſſeſſed to be his own, but that all ſhould be common amongſt Friends. He was furniſhed with legiſlative Knowledge, and a Phyſician that delighted in being able by his Advice and Aſſiſtance to cure his ſick Friends, to whom, whilſt they were well, he took no leſs Pleaſure to philoſophize. However, when Occaſion requir'd, he
judged

judged it as necessary to suspend his Thoughts of the *Ether*, as he expresses it, (1) and assist his City, either by his Wisdom in Council, or by his Valour in War, which in certain Cases he did not disapprove. He also knew how to converse with the Great, and make himself agreeable to the Fair. (2) But what most clearly proves the Excellence of his Morals, is that noble and original Sentiment of his, " That the Whole of human " Virtue may be reduced to speaking " the Truth always, and doing Good to " others." (3)

We find a most eminent Instance of his Prudence, in knowing how to leave his Country, whose Condition did not

pleafe

---

(1) In his Letter, which we have in *Laert.* Sect. 30

(2) That Compliment of his to all the Fair Sex, which we find an Account of from *Timæus* the Historian, in *Laert.* Lib. vIII. 11. deserves our Notice, τας συνοικουσας ανδασι θεων εχ3ηδο ματα, κορας νυμφας ειτα μητερας καλυμειας See also Sect 9 & Sect 11

(3) Ælian Var Hist XII 59 Αληθευειν και ευεργετειν Longin. de Sublim Sect 1 ευεργεσια χαι αληθεια

please him, and to which (by a Fragment of one of his Letters that remains,) we may perceive he did not think himself much obliged. For not having received from his Father, who was a Jewel-Cutter, or Jewel-Merchant, that Nobility by Blood, whereto only this little City had Regard, all his other excellent Qualities were not esteemed there.

And we have another Instance of his great Judgment in chusing *Italy* for his Residence; which was then the most flourishing and happy Part of the World, before the turbulent and rapacious Genius of the *Romans* had Power to lay it waste by its Conquests, as it did a little while after, introducing, together with Slavery, the two inseparable Companions of it, Poverty and Ignorance.

Of this a noble and demonstrative Proof remains, in the Coins of those Countries, and of the neighbouring *Sicily*, minted in those happy Times, whereof a wonderful Abundance is still found, and of a Workmanship excellent beyond all Belief; A certain Sign of the Perfection of Arts, and consequently of their then Opulence; which Coins appear to have failed after those Countries came into the Possession of the *Romans*.

'Twas then, in *Italy*, whilst in this Condition, that *Pythagoras* enjoyed his Glory, beloved universally, respected by the Rich and Powerful: And tho' it was his Fate to lose his Life in a popular Disturbance, as many affirm; or that, as others believe, Circumstances led him to put an End, by a voluntary Abstinence from Food, to his languid and decrepid old Age; certain it is, that his Memory was held in the greatest Reverence; as we may gather from the most eminent Writers both *Greek* and *Latin*, particularly *Cicero*, *Livy*, *Pliny*, and *Plutarch*.

We find, moreover, recorded in these two last Authors, a publick Decree of the Senate of *Rome*, whereby *Pythagoras* (about two Hundred Years after his Death)

Death) was adjudged to be the wisest of all the *Greeks*; and, in consequence of that Title, a Statue was erected to him in the Forum, in Obedience to a certain Oracle of *Apollo*.

In which it is very remarkable, that the same *Pliny* himself wonders he should be preferred to *Socrates*. But if it is considered that *Pythagoras* was also a great Naturalist, and had taught those Things, which *Socrates*, being but little versed in, had entirely neglected, as *Cicero* observes, we shall the more admire the wise Judgment of the *Romans*, who thought that Doctrine less laborious and solid, that did not attempt the precise Exposition and Intelligence of the Nature of material Beings.

There was so great a Mixture of the *Pythagorean* Sentiments, as well philosophical as moral, in the fundamental Constitution of the *Roman* Government, that an ancient Report spread through the World, that King *Numa*, to whom the

D   found-

founding that Constitution was attributed, had been a Pupil of this School, notwithstanding the Repugnancy of such an Opinion to the received Chronology. This Report, tho' supported by the Authority of some old Historians, is, it is certain, very strenuously opposed by *Cicero* and *Livy*, whose Objections are chiefly on account of the *Anacronisms:* But if we reflect seriously, that the original and authentic Monuments being lost, the History and the Chronology of the first Ages of the *Romans* were made up long after, and in many Particulars invented from the Foundation, it will hardly appear strange that a Man of Judgment should chuse to leave such a Controversy undecided, as *Plutarch* has prudently done; it being very difficult to contradict the Reasons, Facts, and Testimonies, which induce us to suspect, either that *Numa* was not of so great Antiquity, or that the Institutions imputed to him were made by wise and careful Persons in much later Times, when *Rome*

appears

appears most plainly to have been a City of *Grecian* Culture. We should also admire the good Taste of *Plato*, who, tho' so great a Follower of the Philosophy of *Socrates*, was nevertheless desirous to come into *Italy*, and there in his Conferences with the *Pythagoreans*, to get that Tincture of Mathematics and true natural Philosophy, which afterwards did him so much Honour.

We ought not indeed to confound with *Pythagoras* all the *Pythagorean* Writers, of which there were many Degrees. The first, and certainly the most learned in the Sciences, as well as the wisest, continued for near two Hundred Years after the Death of their Master; or for nine or ten Generations, as we read in *Laertius*; (1) (and not nineteen, as the printed Copies have it,) the last of this first Sort living at the Time of *Aristotle*. Their School was dissolved by the Change of Government

in

―――――――――――――
(1) Sect. 45, and the Note thereon in the *Menagiana*.

in *Italy*, by the Introduction of the envious Schools of *Socrates* in *Greece*, and by the Obscurity of the *Doric* Dialect, not very common amongst the *Greeks*; whence arose the Difficulty of distinguishing the genuine Writings from the spurious, as *Porphyry* ingeniously observes; to which may be added, that their Doctrines being publish'd by Strangers, and chiefly in an ænigmatical and disguis'd Manner, which, tho' innocent, is always suspected by and disagreeable to those who are unacquainted with it, Calumny and Persecution arose therefrom. Which Persecution of the *Pythagoreans*, as *Polybius* (1) justly remarks, deprived the *Grecian* Cities in *Italy* of their most excellent Men, by which Means they became more exposed to Discord amongst themselves, and to the Violence of the Barbarians their Neighbours.

There arose afterwards in different Countries, and at different Times, a second and

---

(1) Lib. ii. 39.

a third Clafs of *Pythagoreans*, lefs learned and more vifionary; all living after very particular Ways of their own, united into artificial Families in common, either in Cities or in the Country; and which, being full of idolatrous Imaginations and fuperftitious Abftinencies, of Ignorance and Illufions, became defervedly expofed to the Derifion of Mankind; not only of the *Greek* Poets, but of the firft learned and holy Writers of Chriftianity alfo, in whofe Time it appears even thefe laft became extinct.

Diftinguifhing then *Pythagoras* from the *Pythagoreans*, the philofophical School of *Italy*, fubfifting now in our Days, need not be afhamed to own fuch a great Man for its firft Mafter; and among the reft of our Countrymen of *Italy*, it appears, that we *Tufcans* have particular Reafons to refpect his Sentiments and ever-honoured Name; not only on account of that Relation of Family and Original, which many grave ancient Authors

thors have attributed to this Philosopher, with those *Tuscan* Colonies that possessed some of the Islands of *Greece*; but much more, because that from the Time of our Ancestors, the later *Tuscan* Philosophy has followed closely the Method of *Pythagoras*, in making Geometry the Foundation of all other Studies; and that the establishing three of the principal Doctrines of the old *Pythagoreans*, that of the Roundness of the Earth, its Motion about the Sun, and the Nullity of the Generation of Animals from Corruption, has done so much Honour to the Memory of our three famous Countrymen, *Americus Vespasianus*, *Galileo*, and *Redi*.

And yet more should the *Tuscan* Philosophers who study Physic esteem the Opinions of *Pythagoras*, with relation to what concerns their Art, because he was, as *Celsus* observes, the first and most illustrious of all the Professors of Philosophy who had applied themselves to that Study, and because the *Italian* Physicians

of

of the Age of *Pythagoras*, and of those Countries where he had propagated his Doctrines most, were (as (1) *Herodotus* the Father of the *Grecian* History attests) the first of all *Greece*, and the most sought after. And because the *Pythagorean* Physicians were also the first that dissected Animals, and register'd particular Experiments of their Medicines, for which *Alcmeon* and *Acron* were so justly celebrated.

But this same intrinsic Goodness of the medical Opinions of *Pythagoras* will always give judicious Enquirers a great Idea of his Penetration into the Nature of the human Body. Those who do not form a Judgment of Things easily, or on slight Grounds, but by long Study and philosophical Labour have acquired a true Knowledge of Physic by numberless Observations on distemper'd Bodies, cannot but admire the Certainty and Importance of the *Pythagorean* Doctrine, on the alternate Increase and Remission of most Distempers

(1) Lib. iii. P. 137, & H. S.

pers upon every third Day, together with the most remarkable Phœnomena that attend our Bodies, in septenary Periods; without entering into the Necessity of supposing, as it appears those later *Pythagoreans* have done, that *Celsus* and *Galen* were so much surprized at it.

These we may with a safe Conscience neglect; and, as it has been said, it would be wrong to confound them with *Pythagoras* himself, who was much above all such Follies, it being far more reasonable to believe, that wise Man, who was as well assured of the Truth of the Phœnomena as we are, was likewise no less capable of understanding the true Reason thereof, founded on the Elasticity or natural Contraction of the Fibres whereof the human Body is composed, and upon their finite Power of being extended, and which must therefore be confined within some certain Bounds.

A Belief that Health is the principal

Part or Basis of human Happiness, (1) and that it depends on a Harmony, that is, a Correspondence of the several Motions with the Powers that produce them: And that it consists immediately in the Permanence of Figure, as Distemper does in the Alteration of it. That by the original Formation at our Birth, Events happening afterwards successively in the Body, were determined according to the Combination of exterior Causes. That the two chiefest Instruments of Life are the Brain and the Heart. That the liquid Humours of the human Body are distinguished into three different Substances, according to the Difference of their Densities, *viz.* Blood, Water, (whether *Serum* or *Lymph*) and Vapour. That there are three Kinds of Vessels, Nerves, Arteries, and Veins. That the prolific animated Matter, by its Application to the Embrionic Body, puts its Blood in Motion, whereof the Parts af-

---

(1) Schol antiq de Aristoph N v 609

terwards form themselves, even the most fleshy, solid, and long. These and such other like Things, being Sparks as it were of the best medical Theory, we meet with in the Extract *Laertius* has given of (1) the Doctrines of *Pythagoras*, from the Books of that learned *Alexander* the *Greek*, who lived in the Time of *Sylla*, and who by his vast Erudition acquired the Sirname of *Polyhistor*. Which Opinions, so consistent with Truth, and received at this Day in the most enlighten'd Schools, produce in thinking Readers, that pleasing Satisfaction which results from observing the Agreement of the Thoughts of great Men in all Ages and in all Countries.

The Preference then which the *Pythagorean* Practice of Physic gave to a Regimen in Diet, above all other Remedies, makes the Sagacity of those Professors highly esteemed, by all that know how tedious the Experiments are, whereby that noble Incredulity in the Virtues of Drugs is at last acquir'd,

(1) Sect 28, &c. Nov Verf (og.

quir'd, which has so remarkably distinguish'd a few Physicians from the many and vulgar Practitioners of that Art. In this Branch of Physic, as *Jamblicus* informs us, (1) the *Pythagoreans* were the most exact: Measuring the Quantity of Victuals, and of Drink, of Exercise, and of Rest, by Rule; determining the Choice and Manner of preparing what they allowed, (a Thing neglected by others) and making Use more willingly of external than other Medicines: Paying but a small Regard to Pharmacy, and in their Surgery being very sparing of the Knife, and universally abhorring the Use of Fire.

But what shall we say of that other noble Invention which we owe to *Pythagoras*, and which is one of the most powerful, and at the same time one of the most safe, and most universal Medicines, that Human Industry has ever to this Day been able to find out, however it remain'd neglected for so many Ages, tho' a fatal

Inadver-

(1) Vit de Pythag. 1. 29.

Inadvertency, till in this happy Age it was at last again brought into the Use of philosophical Medicine? I mean the *Pythagorean* Diet, which consisted (1) in the free and universal Use of every Thing that is vegetable, tender and fresh, which requires little or no Preparation to make it fit to eat, such as Roots, Leaves, Flowers, Fruits and Seeds: And in a general Abstinence from every Thing that is animal, whether it be fresh or dried, Bird, Beast, or Fish.

Milk and Honey made up part of this Diet: Eggs, on the contrary, were excluded. Their Drink was to be the purest Water; neither Wine nor any vinous Liquor. The Exactness of the Diet might, indeed, sometimes, as Occasion requir'd, be departed from, by mingling some very moderate Portion of animal Food therewith, provided it were of young and tender

---

(1) We find this Diet call'd by various Names among the Antients, Ἄψυχος βίος ὁ τῶν Πυθαγορικῶν Πομφαγία, Βοτανοφαγία by *Hesychius* Vita inanimata The Herb Diet Ποιηφαγέειν by *Herodotus* Cœna terrestris multis oleribus by *Plautus*

der Meat, fresh and sound, and that of the muscular Parts rather than the Entrails (1).

From this only faithful Exposition of the *Pythagorean* Diet, we may immediately see that it agrees with the best Rules in Physic, drawn from the most exact Knowledge the Moderns have acquir'd of the Nature of the Human Body, and of the alimental Substances. Insomuch that whoever thinks of the Matter with any Sagacity, can hardly doubt but that *Pythagoras* himself, the first Inventor of this Diet, had Health principally in View, as well as that so-much-to-be-desir'd Tranquility of Mind, that is a Consequence of it, and that results from a more easy Supply of our Wants, a more uniform Calm of the Humours, and a constant Habit of suppressing, by Temperance, our most noxious Desires.

Which Supposition appears much more suitable to his Wisdom, than to imagine,
that

---

(1) We find all these Particulars chiefly in *Laertius* and *Porphyrius*.

that he chose such a Diet, because he believed from his Heart a Transmigration of Souls, a Doctrine he seems to have made Use of as a plausible Reason for his Practice, finding himself, as we have hinted, under a Necessity of speaking according to the Capacity of the People, which People (he well knew) did neither understand nor regard the true and natural Reasons. He was fully sensible that the Faculty of Thinking, and the Principle of voluntary Motion, which every Man finds within himself, cannot be accounted for by any Knowledge we have of dead Matter, or by mechanical Principles. And therefore he admitted that *Egyptian* Hypothesis of the Nature of the Soul, dressing it up in Fables according to the Custom of that Nation. (1) This Hypothesis is indeed certainly not true, nor conformable to the clearer Lights we now have, but it has had at least in the World this true Merit, that it has led to the introducing into the Schools of the

Philo-

---

(1) Herodot l. ii.

Philosophers, the Seeds of so interesting a Doctrine as that of the Immortality of the Soul.

But that *Pythagoras* did not admit among his secret Opinions the passing of Souls from one Body to another, and retaining their Ideas and Identity, we may gather from the Authority of *Timæus, Plato's Pythagorean* Master, in that elegant Book of his which by great Chance has been preserved; wherein he with sufficient Sincerity, in his *Doric* Dialect, expresses his real Meaning (1) in the following Words:

"We restrain Mankind by false Reasons, says he, if they will not let us guide them by the true. Whence arises the Necessity of talking of those strange Punishments of Souls, as if they passed out of one Body into another."

Who can ever imagine that *Pythagoras*, whose Opinion was that even Plants are animated, was not aware that living

---

(1) Towards the End, τὰς ψυχὰς ἀπείργομες ψευδέσι λογοις ὁκα μὴ ἄγηται ἀλαθέσι, λέγοιντο δ' ἀναγκαῖι και τιμωρίαι ξέναι ὡς μετενδοκείαν τᾶν ψυχᾶν, &c.

Creatures could not possibly feed on Minerals, nor consequently be otherwise supported than by eating Plants? Whence his Doctrine of Abstinence would have been in its own Nature impossible and foolish. And indeed, that his Doctrine of the Transmigration of Souls was only a specious Reason to make his medical Advice go down with People, since that Truths drawn from natural and philosophical Arguments are only satisfactory to the Wise, that is, to a very small Part of Mankind, was also the Opinion of some among the Antients: As we may gather from *Laertius* who uses the following Words (1):

" The Sameness of the Nature of the
" Soul was indeed a Pretence for the for-
" bidding the eating of Animals: But the
" Truth was, that he intended by such a
" Prohibition to accustom Men to con-
" tent themselves with such a Diet as was
" every where to be found with Ease,
" (which they might eat without dressing)
" and

(1) Section XIII.

" and with drinking only pure Water; all
" which is highly conducive both to the
" Health of the Body, and the Alacrity
" of the Mind (1)."

Which Sentiment it also appears that *Plutarch* had, who, in his Treatise on eating Flesh, (2) after collecting many philosophical, medical, and moral Reasons to disswade Mankind from such a Custom, or from the Abuse of it at least, excuses himself for not making Use of the Reasons of *Pythagoras*, which he calls full of Mystery, and resembles to the hidden Machines that moved the Scenes at the Theatre, and by way of Allegory mentions, on that Occasion, the poetical Imaginations of *Empedocles*. And this manner of understanding, consistently with Reason, such

---

(1) In the printed Copy it says, ἄπυρα, which is equal to the ἄνευ πυρός, that is, without Fire, or without much Preparation of Cookery. The *Latin* Translation of the finest Edition of *Meibomius* gives for it, *Ea quæ anima carent*, which is a manifest Mistake. The old Translation by *Ambrosius* is more faithful, *Quibus igni ad coquendum opus non esset*, and it is still better in that of *Aldobrandinus*, which says, *Cibis minime coctis*.

(2) Opusc. vol. III περὶ σαρκῶν p. 1833.

a Doctrine, in Appearance incredible, of a Man otherwise exceeding wise and cautious, is render'd yet much the more probable from the Authority of many old Writers, who assert, as may be seen particularly in *Laertius*, *Gellius*, and *Athenæus*, that *Pythagoras* eat, himself, and advised others to eat, from Time to Time, without Scruple, Chickens, Kids, tender Pigs, sucking Calves, and Fish, nor did he abhor Beans, as the Vulgar thought, or any other kind of Pulse. And perhaps the Contradictions of the most serious Authors upon this Subject may be reconcil'd, by a Supposition, that he only rejected such Things as were hard and dry, contenting himself with those that were fresh and tender. If we then examine, with Diligence and Judgment, all that we find on this Subject dispers'd in a great many Books, we may understand clearly that the Intention of this Philosopher was only to cure Diseases and Corpulency, as well as gross Habits and clouding of the Senses and Understanding,

by

by the Use of a sparing Diet upon chosen kinds of Food, and a total Abstinence from Wine.

True it is, that certain particular Abstinences, similar to those of *Pythagoras*, were formerly made Use of by several Nations, and especially by the *Egyptians*, from whom it is probable that Philosopher might take his first Hint; since it is manifest that he took a Pleasure to intermix in his own manner, and with his own Thoughts, many of the Sentiments of that learned, but mysterious Nation.

One of these Abstinences, rigorously and universally observed in *Egypt*, was that from Beans, as *Herodotus* observes: (1) Which we find propagated afterwards amongst the *Greeks* and *Romans*, principally by the Priests of *Jupiter*, and *Ceres*, and of their other false and absurd Deities (2). But by whatever Means it came into the Head of *Pythagoras* to propose an Abstinency

---

(1) Lib. ii.
(2) Paus. lib. viii. 15. Porphyr. de Abstin. lib. iv. Gell. x. 15. Fest. v. *Fabam*, &c.

nency from Beans, it is now plain, from the general Senſe of all the antient Writers, that this Prohibition of his was allegorical, and that it would be now a vain Undertaking to attempt finding out the literal Senſe of it, ſince thoſe who knew it were ſo induſtrious to keep it ſecret.

And as we find, on the other hand, that *Pythagoras* made no Difficulty of eating them, and that he extended his Prohibition concerning Food even to other kinds of Pulſe, as alſo to old Cocks, plowing Oxen, and many other Subſtances of a like hard glutinous Conſiſtence; it ſeems much more reaſonable to ſuppoſe, that the ſymbolical Prohibition of Beans was ſomething entirely different, of an important and ſecret Signification; and that the real Abſtinences intended, were indeed firſt preſcribed by others before him, and for other Ends; (1) but that they were by him firſt of all adopted and promoted as medical and moral Councils, under

(1) Laert viii 33 ἀπεχεσθαι ὧν παρα κελευον ται καὶ οἱ τὰς τελετὰς ἐν τοῖς ἱεροῖς ἐπιτελοῦν σεν.

der whatever Covering he was then pleas'd to give them an Authority.

And his Knowledge may appear wonderful, in that he forbid, in Flesh itself, that of carnivorous Animals above all other Kinds; and, for the same Reason, that of Wild Boars, and what was taken in Hunting, with most Sorts of Fishes; and in all Animals whatever, those Parts that are the most tender and delicate, such as the Glands, the Viscera, and the Eggs: Being aware, as *Clemens Alexandrinus* observes, of their being the least wholesome, from their very strong and pungent Effluvia, which in the modern Schools would be rather term'd their more abounding in oleaginous and volatile Salts. His two only Meals in a Day, equivalent to our Collations, were for the most Part of Bread only, but his last Meal, which we should call a Supper, was in sufficient Abundance; and his drinking at such times some Wine, not in the Day-time only, but at Evenings,

in

in decent Company at Table, his Cloaths that were white and extremely (1) clean, and which he chang'd every Day under the Colour of Religion; his prefering those made of vegetable Matter (2) to those made of animal Substances, which he knew to be more attractive of the moist and unwholesome Effluvia of the Air; (3) the Delight he took in Music, when separated from all that was vicious or offensive, (4) his pleasant and learned Conversation among his Friends, his Care of the Neatness of his Person, with the frequent Use of Baths, not public and noisy, but private and quiet at Home, together with his other agreeable and genteel Manners, mention'd in all the

Writers

(1) Diodor. Sicul &c.
(2) *Apul.* Apol p. 64 and *Porc. Jambl.* c 21. *Philostr.* Vit. Ap. viii 3 He makes the same Objection as *Laertius*, that Linnen was not yet introduced in the Place where *Pythagoras* dwelt, but it is certain, that the Use of Linnen Cloths and of the finest Cotton, was then very frequent in *Egypt*, whither that Manufacture was brought from *India* So that *Pythagoras*, and all the other *Greeks* who made Use of it, might have it from *Egypt*. Vid. also *Ferrar. d re vest.* p ii lib 4 c. 1 & 12
(3) *Jacob Keil* Medicin statica 178 plus attrahunt vessels e partibus animalium compositæ quam quæ e vegetabilibus conficiuntur, &c.
(4) Jambl. 29

Writers that have treated of his private Life, shew that this worthy Man was in all his ways very different from what he has been thought by those that have represented him as harsh, austere, and horribly superstitious.

That Precept of his, which we find recorded in all the Writers of his Life, concerning the not destroying or hurting any domestic or fruit-bearing Plants, or any Animal but what is venomous and noxious; with the Account of his buying Fish, and after having well consider'd their different Forms on the River's Bank, returning them to the Water again, (1) must make us imagine him (if I am not mistaken) very far from that ridiculous Superstition which is vulgarly attributed to him; and which we see, by other Instances, he from his Heart abhorred. (2) These Things rather serve to inform us, that he was full of that delicate Spirit of innocent Curiosity, proper

---

(1) Plutarch & Apuleius.
(2) Besides the Writers of his Life, we find it in many Places, Liv. xl. 29. Plin. xiii. 13. Plutar. Num. p. 136.

per to true Naturalists, and of that reasonable Desire of preserving, as much as possible, all organiz'd Bodies whatever; which, if of no other Use, have at least that of furnishing us with an agreeable and curious Entertainment: And that he had in him a strong Feeling of that provident Humanity, so contrary to the childish, restless, and destructive Inclination we see in too many, of pulling to Pieces and spoiling, for the most trifling Purposes, the beautiful and useful Productions of Nature.

How effectual then this *Pythagorean* Diet is, towards obtaining the End for which, as has been said, it was principally intended by its Author; that is, for preserving the present Health of the Body, or for the restoring that which is lost, may easily be understood by whoever will but consider the Nature and Faculties of our Bodies, as also of the Aliments which sustain them; not according to the poetical Imaginations of the barbarous Schools, but according to the secure Lights that have been obtained

in

in our Time by the Study of anatomical and mechanical Medicine, natural History, and experimental Philosophy, of which true and rational Chymistry makes no inconsiderable Part.

These Lights have finally made us understand, that Life and Health consist in the perpetual and equable Motion of a large Mass of Liquid distributed through innumerable continued Channels, which dividing into Trunks and Branches, are reduc'd in their Extremities to an inexpressible Degree of Minuteness, and to a Multiplicity without Number. The capital Trunks of these Channels, which are as it were their Basis, are only two; of a different Fabrick and Nature, situated nearly in the Center of the Body, and conjoin'd to the Heart: And their Terminations or Extremities open, some of them upon the outward Surface of the Body, or into some Cavities within it, and others of them communicate, and inosculate together, the Extremities of one Sort into thofe of the other.

And as the grand Mafs of the Fluid is carried, and runs continually through thefe Channels, one of the two Trunks, which is called an Artery, with all the innumerable Ramifications depending on it, muft carry the faid Fluid from the Cavity of the Heart, by the Force there given it, and by the continued Action of the Channel itfelf, partly to the Surface of the Body, where it is diffipated into its Pores; partly to the internal Cavities, where it is depofited; and laftly, the other Part to the fineft and utmoft Ramifications of the other Channel, which is called a Vein; where by the direct Impulfe of the continually following Fluid, and by the lateral Preffure of the Veffels, it is finally re-conducted by a contrary Motion to the Heart again.

By this Diftribution it is manifeft, that if the arterial Veffels fhould fend back to the venal the entire Mafs of the Fluid, fuch such a Course might last, and go on as far as depended only on the Quantity, but as only one Part of it passes from the Arteries into the Veins, its Course could not long be maintain'd, was it not that the Veins receive a continual new Addition of fresh Fluid, which they take in, by such of their Extremities as open into the Cavity of a large Bag or Channel, from the Mass or Mixture of the Aliments that are introduced thither from without.

Thus the internal Course of the Fluids, which we call Life, is continual in all living Beings, that is, in all natural organical Bodies, be they Plants or Animals: With this principal Difference, that Plants, always fix'd to the Ground, receive their Supply of new Liquids (by their Veins opening upon the Surfaces of their Roots) from that Part of the Earth which totally surrounds them from without: Whereas Animals, who have the Power of transporting their Bodies into various Places, sustain their Lives no otherwise than by introducing, from time to time, into a Cavity within themselves, that is, into the Stomach and Intestines, a kind (as it were) of portable Earth, or a Mass of various Matter well mingled and well moisten'd, from which they draw, by their radical Veins, inward to the Heart, the incorporable Moisture with which they are nourished.

And as this Fluid which moves in the Human Body, and of which a sufficient Quantity ought thus to be supplied by Food, is not of a simple Nature like Water, besides the Disorders which may be produc'd by the Obstruction of its Motion, or the Decay of the Channels in which it moves, there are also others that depend on its Qualities and its Composition. Hence arises the Necessity of a Choice in the Subject of our Food, from which all Minerals are universally to be excluded, as no way capable of being changed into our Substance, but much more

more likely, by their Hardness and Weight, to lacerate our tender Organs, than to be by them separated and digested.

A considerable Quantity of Salt, either marine or similar to it, is, indeed, taken into the Body with our Food by way of Seasoning; but no Part thereof is converted into our Substance, it being all dissolv'd and discharg'd again out of the Body, or that very little Part which remains unchang'd, is in a manner of no effect. Water, which is taken into the Body in great Quantities, either pure or mingled with other Matters, may conduce much towards maintaining the Course of our Fluids, and even render liquid some of the solid Particles that have been left in the Vessels, by serving them as a Vehicle, and may thereby (tho' indirectly) serve to nourish our Bodies, for some Days, without any other Food; but Water never entirely loses its own proper Qualities, nor changes itself into their Substance, how intimately soever

soever it becomes mingled with our constituent Particles.

All other Substances appertaining to the fossil Kingdom, remain entirely excluded from human Food. The Doubt then lies only between Vegetables and Animals, which of these two Substances are most likely to become proper and useful Matter for our Bodies. *Plutarch* long since (in his Treatise against eating Flesh) has made it a Question, whether such kind of Aliment was natural to Man, that is, suitable to the Fabrick of his Body. And it is now about a hundred Years, as we find in the Letters of *Gassendus*, since this Matter was disputed very particularly amongst the Learned, who observed that all other Animals were, by their constant Habit and Manner of Life, depending on the natural Structure and Action of their Organs of Digestion, readily distinguish'd into those that feed on the Fruits of the Earth, and the rapacious and carnivorous: Whereupon

upon as the Queſtion could not be decided this way, or by any Arguments drawn from natural Hiſtory, the ſame Queſtion has ſince been again propoſed and demonſtrated, by that eminent Mathematician Dr. *Wallis*, and that diligent Anatomiſt Dr. *Tyſon*, as we read in the Philoſophical Tranſactions of *England*, (1) from the greater Analogy in the Fabrick of the Paſſages of the Aliment, and of the Organs of Digeſtion in Men, with thoſe of ſuch Animals as feed on vegetable Diet, moſt of which, like Men, are furniſh'd with a Gut *Colon*, whereof moſt of the Carnivorous are deſtitute.

But leaving theſe Reflections, which may appear too far fetch'd, we ſhould rather conſider, that moſt of the Animals which ſerve for human Food feed on Vegetables, except only ſome few Birds and Fiſhes; from whence it finally appears, that the ultimate Matter of the two chief kinds of Aliment is almoſt the ſame in its firſt Compo-

Composition, that is, always vegetable, and coming originally from the Earth. Thus, for the most part, what fixes and unites itself to the Body of Man, either from the one or the other sort of Aliment, is really nothing else but some of the solid and purest Earth.

But the Difference principally consists, in that the fresh Parts of Plants, being of a much tenderer Texture than those of Animals, are therefore much easier to be seperated, (from the lesser Course of their Cohesion and internal Glew) and so yield more easily to the dividing Power of our Organs. The tender and fresh Parts of Plants abound with Water, and that sort of Salts, which by Reason of their Taste, and Non-evaporation by Fire, before they are dissolv'd, we call acid and fix'd: To the Mixture of which, with a moderate oily and vegetable Fluid, is owing their incorporating and dissolving Juice. Of this Juice Animal Food is destitute, as it is also entirely of the said acid and fixed Salts,

but

but it abounds, on the contrary, with such as are apt to become, with a certain Degree of Heat, of an alcaline and volatile Nature, and to occasion, by their Mixture, the greatest Disposition in our Liquids to an ultimate and totally mortiferous Dissolution. And on the lesser Quantity and less perfect oily Quality of fresh Vegetables, depends a Disposition in the Juices from them produc'd, less apt, without Comparison, to receive those superlative Degrees of Heat in their greatest and most intimate Agitations, whilst they are carried about in the Blood: For Experience shews, that no Liquid is found in all Nature more ready than Oil to receive or retain the Force of Fire, whether apparent or latent: from whatever Substance such Oil is extracted; altho' that of Animals seems yet more prompt and efficacious than all others.

How subtle our vital Fluid must be, is then manifest, from its forming itself, gradually and finally, into a Substance, fit for insensible Transpiration, and into that spirituous Air that exhales continually, both within and without, from every living Body. In this Subtilty and Facility of our Liquid's being distributed into the innumerable Ramifications of the Vessels, consists its Fluidity, without which those Particles that are hard and weighty would be deposited in some Places, and would by that Means fill up the Cavities which ought to be kept empty and always open. From the Addition then of an aqueous, oily, and saline Juice, which the Chymists call saponaceous, to the Substance of that innocent and sweet Soil, with which Vegetable Aliments, as has been said, are so plentifully endued, arises that so necessary and perfect Commixture of the dissimilar Parts of our Blood, and especially of those two most copious Fluids that so constantly avoid, and are so difficult to incorporate with each other, (I mean Water and Oil) and whose Separation, when it happens within us, produces such pernicious Effects.

fects. And the much smaller Quantity of the oleaginous Liquor that is found in fresh Vegetables, in Comparison of what is found in Flesh, not only prevents the Formation of a too tenacious Gluten, but also of that Vapour, which, rising with the Increase of our bodily Heat, when the fat and saline Particles grow volatile, becomes itself, at last, venomous, and even productive of Pestilence.

I have always named fresh Vegetables, because the dry'd ones have almost all the bad Qualities of Animal Food, particularly as their earthy and oleaginous Particles are too strongly coherent together. We should thus likewise exclude all aromatic Spices, and substitute in their stead, the green Tops of odoriferous and agreeable Herbs; we should reject old Pulse, and all farinaceous and oily Seeds, unless they are by Art well pounded, and mingled and dissolved with other useful Matters. We may say the same thing of dry'd Fruits, and of whatever else is preserv'd in various ways,

ways, and which compos'd the dry'd Diet of the Antients: the which, however it may have been commended as an Instance of Hardiness, was not perhaps of the greatest Advantage to their Healths.

Honey, tho' gather'd from Bees, is reckon'd amongst the vegetable Juices: Being preserv'd for some Time in certain little Bags within their Bodies, it is discharg'd from thence into their Hives, from whence we make ourselves Masters of it. It is collected from the most refin'd and most perfect Juices of Plants, separated from the Mass which moves within them, and united into those little Lumps that are deposited at the Bottom of the Leaves of the Flowers, and which *Malpighi* has (1) observ'd and describ'd. Sugar is also the natural Product of Plants, tho' extracted from them by the Assistance of Art. Both these Matters are oily and saline, and of a wonderfully attenuating, detersive, and saponaceous Virtue, especially when mixt
with

(1) Anatom Plant Tab 29

with other Food, and particularly with Water, and are not hurtful, as vulgarly believ'd, but exceedingly useful and good.

Milk is good also in a remarkable manner, and principally that of Animals which feed on Grass and Herbs. This Liquor, tho' labour'd and compos'd by the Animal Organs, of the Juice of their Aliment, and of some of their own proper Juices; and altho' pass'd through their Bowels, and through their least arterial Channels, has not, nevertheless, lost all the Qualities of Vegetables, retaining principally that wholsome Disposition of becoming acid; nor is it wholly changed into an Animal Nature, but has acquir'd by Trituration, a Fluidity and Commixture, whereby it has obtained a greater Aptitude to be readily converted into our Substance: Being besides agreeable to all our Senses when fresh milked and at a proper Time; and therefore, in the Judgment of the most excellent Physicians of all Ages, it is thought to be a most light, good, and simple Aliment, and singular

gular in its Nature, by reason of its middle Temperament between vegetable and animal Food: Wherefore it is most wrongfully despised and dreaded by the unexperienc'd Part of Mankind

Much pure Water with Milk makes the best of Mixture; it was used and praised even by *Hippocrates*, who attributes the Invention of it to *Pitocles*, a Physician more antient than himself (1), who employ'd it with much Advantage, particularly as a safe Means of restoring those who were too lean and extenuated. A little Wine with much Milk, which some Nations use to this Day, has also the Authority of the Antients in its Favour; tho' it does not appear so proper for Medicine, as, with convenient Seasoning, it may be made perhaps for the Delicacy of the Table: And yet much less reasonable and less pleasant will appear the mixing of Broth, or other unctuous Liquids, or of some savory Substances with Milk, as it never can
stand

( ) Epidem v 55 & vii 48

stand in need of bettering its Qualities, tho' it may sometimes want its Fluidity to be increased, which may at all Times be done by its Mixture with common Water.

And because either by standing, or by Agitation, or by boiling, or by the Mixture of certain acid Juices of Plants or Materials in the Act of boiling, Milk readily separates into those three well known Substances of Cream or Butter, Whey, and Cheese: It is easy to comprehend, that the Whey, by its Fluidity and Temperature, is a very good Medicine in some Cases; especially when given in such large Quantities as five, or six, or more Pounds a Day, as the Antients gave it, and the Butter, tho' oily, may, in a moderate Dose, be admitted into our Victuals, provided it has no offensive Rancidity, the Cheese also is very good when it is fresh and new, but that which is hard and dry, and which is, by too long keeping, become acrid and biting to the Taste, having acquir'd bad Qualities not suitable to this our Design, should be used

but

but rarely, and then very sparingly, only as Seasoning; and the same Caution and Forbearance should be used also as to Eggs.

The vegetable Juices taken from some Parts of Plants, which, by the Means of Fermentation are brought to become those known Liquors which we call Wines, Beers, and Meads, and much more the Spirits thence extracted, are quite opposite to the Intentions of the *Pythagorean* Diet: because by fermenting they have acquir'd a contrary Nature, and instead of dissolving, and continually more and more liquifying and diminishing the Cohesion and glutinous Quality of our vital Fluid, they serve, on the contrary, only to increase it. Whence arises their present Faculty of re-invigorating, and increasing the Motion and Heat of our Bodies, besides their singular Power of so readily offending the Nerves, and disturbing their Operations, according to the different Degrees or Progressions of their venomous Efficacy, to produce a so-much-desir'd, tho' a false Alacrity

Alacrity and Delirium, Forgetfulness and Sluggishness; which Effects many call sweet and amiable, but the *Pythagorean* looks upon them in a very different Light, and knows how often those seeming Pleasures are attended with Palsies, with Apoplexies, and with Death; which but too soon succeed those temporary Gratifications of the Mind, produc'd only by Liquors so fermented.

Entirely different from Wine is that Liquor which may be form'd therefrom, but by a second Fermentation, which we call Vinegar. This, having precipitated its most gross and unctuous Parts, becomes limpid and subtle, penetrating and volatile, and therefore apt to insinuate and mingle itself intimately with our still oily Fluids, and by such Means to prevent, or mitigate at least, that worst of Changes which is frequently made within us by the Force of our vital Heat and Motion, and what is commonly known by the Names of *putrid Acrimony*, *Rancidity*, or *Alkalescence*.

Hence Vinegar is a great Refrigerative in acute Fevers, produced either by the internal Stimulus of the human Juices then made alkaline, or by some venomous Quality, introduced from without; and ever since the Time of *Hippocrates* it has been of great and salutary Service in Medicine and Surgery. It expels Drunkenness, Sleepiness, and Weakness, by agreeably invigorating the Nerves, to which it is a singular Friend. In all Pestilences, and especially in our last, the very great Efficacy of Vinegar was evident, notwithstanding the bad Mixture of a great Number of other Medicines of a contrary Nature then made Use of (1).

And since a little of the best Wine in a great deal of Water forms a Liquor very ready to turn acid by the internal Heat of the Body, that is, perhaps, the Reason why an Abundance of such Drink has prov'd salutiferous, in some habitual, and sometimes even in acute Fevers among the Antients,

as

---

(1) Rondinelli relazione del contagione del 1630.

as we find particularly in the Writings of *Hippocrates*: And Experience shews us, that in many Cases it is so with us also.

Of such, and still greater Value, are the acid and fresh Juices of sowr and other Fruits: Wherefore, it is no wonder, if some have made Use of them, as an agreeable and powerful Remedy against malignant and pestilential Fevers. Nor is this a new Invention, for amongst ourselves, it is now about an hundred Years since such a Virtue in Verjuice was observed by *Famianus Michelini*, who was Reader of Mathematics in the School of *Pisa*, (2) and who having been a Scholar of the great *Borelli*, was, on that Account, delighted greatly with Anatomy and Physic. Some of his Trials were made very happily in *Pisa*, at the Time when malignant Fevers raged there, and when the greatest Part of those that were seiz'd with them, if treated in the usual Methods, died. His Secret (as

---

(2) Known in the World by his Treatise, entitled, *Della direzione de Fiumi*, printed at *Florence* 1664

I find in his original Writings) consisted in drinking largely of Lemon and Orange Juice, or in some Cases even of Verjuice with a great deal of Water: and in taking no other Food but the Crumb of Bread, boiled or sop'd in fair Water. Supposing always that this Care was taken from the Beginning of the Distemper, this Method was certainly extremely good and judicious, and deserved not to be derided, as it was by his lazy Rivals; nor to be made a Secret to Men of Learning, who were, even at that Time, capable of comprehending its Consonancy to the philosophical Truths of Medicine, to the Experience of all preceding Ages, and to the Authorities of the most approved Masters.

It does not then appear that *Michelini* supposed, that the Product of any acid Mineral Spirits, which are rather hurtful to the human Body, were any way equivalent to vegetable Acids; though it is evident, he was not aware of the Universality of the like Virtues in all acid vegetable Juices,

Juices, whether of Fruits or Herbs, and particularly of Vinegar: insomuch, that perhaps among all the vulgar Errors of Medicine, the most pernicious and opposite to Experience and good Reasoning, is the Supposition, that acid Juices are mischievous. We should indeed give them (next to Water) the Praise of being the most certain and universal Remedies; as they are, at the same time, both agreeable and very resolvent; whereas Coagulation produces the most fatal Effects of all Distempers, as the anatomical Knife well demonstrates. The *Pythagoreans* then had great Reason for their Esteem of Vinegar, and of all the fresh acid Juices of the several Sorts of Fruits and Herbs; and to prefer them to any aromatic, fat, or spirituous Correctives and Seasonings.

Oil, tho' vegetable, and simply extracted, as it is a Liquor entirely fat, and therefore very apt to acquire a hurtful Rancidness in the alimentary Channels, if not soon changed by the digestive Powers,
should

should not only be chosen the sweetest that can be had, and so the farthest from its rancid Corruption, but also be us'd sparingly and seldom, and mix'd with acid Juices, for the seasoning of Foods otherwise very wholesome in themselves.

Experience, join'd with sagacious Reasoning, has, in a like Manner, determin'd us to chuse out of the vast Variety of vegetable Matters which the Earth affords, those only, which, either being spontaneously the best of their Kinds, or render'd so by Art, have a tender and brittle Texture, with an aqueous Juice, either insipid, or sweet, or agreeably acid, or milky and bitterish, and in some Cases perfectly bitter and sharp; and that either have no Smell, or else one that is sweet, or sometimes even strong and penetrating: diminishing or increasing each of these Qualities, according as there is Need, by boiling and mixing them with Preparations that are proper. From whence it happens, that if we would reckon up exactly all the Vegetables

getables that afford us either their Roots, or their whole Bodies, or their Leaves and Blossoms, or their Flowers, or their Fruits, their Seeds or their Juices, for the Substance of our Food, or for a Seasoning to it, we should not make Use of a hundred of those Kinds of Plants, whereof there are above a Thousand known in the present System of Botany.

And there would still be much fewer, were we to make a more rigorous Choice according to the Principle here laid down; whereby we should entirely exclude all those vegetable Substances that are of an invigorating and pungent Nature, and those which afford the most solid Nourishment. We should then, with the scrupulous Abstinence of the *Egyptians*, avoid Onions, Garlick, and all the bulbous Roots, and forbear all dry Fruits, Nuts, and all the hardest Kinds of Seeds; admitting only Corn, (which serves for making Bread, or to give a Body to Water, or Broth, wherein it is boiled,) and some of the most delicate

licate Pulse, now and then, for Variety, either fresh and tender, or even dryed, but notwithstanding dissolved and mingled with the softest Herbs, or with some of the watery Fruits. Thus *Taurus*, a Philosopher of *Athens*, and a great Admirer of *Pythagoras*, as we find in *Aulus Gellius*, (who had often been at his Table) (1) used to do by Lentils and Gourds. Whence we shall easily find, that the Plants which can satisfy the Needs, and even Delicacies, of a *Pythagorean* Table, throughout the whole Year, scarce amount to the Number of Forty; all of which, excepting that which produces Sugar, are usually cultivated amongst us in our Fields and Gardens; and those which are the most common, are also the most wholesome.

Such then being the Nature and Qualities of the selected Aliments which compose a fresh vegetable Diet, it should not appear wonderful to any, if by that alone,
con-

(1) Lib. xvii c. 8.

constantly us'd for some Length of Time, and tempered as the Discretion of a wise Philosopher shall direct, when there may be Occasion, by a Mixture of some few, and those chosen Kinds of Flesh, and especially Flesh boiled with tender and fresh Herbs, either sour, or lactiferous and sweet, sometimes also odorous and bitter, we may remove, with Ease, many Infirmities, otherwise invincible by human Art: prevent others, and universally dispose the Body to be less susceptible of the Danger of morbid Infections.

In the *Pythagorean* is included a *Milk Diet* also; that is, living entirely upon Milk, as all young Animals do, and as it is said some whole Nations did anciently, and still do even in our own Times; this Milk Diet was introduced throughout all *Europe*, for the Cure of some Diseases, and especially of the Gout and Rheumatism, about the Middle of the last Century, by the Sagacity and Experience of a gouty

Physician of *Paris:* (1) tho' it does not wholly want the Example and Authority of the Ancients, and chiefly of *Hippocrates, Celsus, Pliny,* and many others, among which, (at least of those whom we have any Remains of,) it appears that *Aretæus* was the first who made Use of Milk alone, in some Distempers, without any other Aliment: arguing with good Reason for its Sufficiency and Salubrity, from the Custom of whole Nations who liv'd upon that only.

The Opinion of a Milk-Diet for the Gout was greatly confirm'd, for about fifty Years together, by various Experiments made in *England;* where it was soon after discover'd, that even living, for a few Weeks only, on some fresh and wholesome Herbs, without any other Food, had the same Effect in that troublesome Disorder; (2) and the like Reputation was there at last extend-

(1) *See* Griesel de cura lactis in Atritide. Vien Austr. 1670, p 179

(2) Dr Fr Slare gives a Proof of this in Turnips, in a Letter printed along with a Treatise of Dr Geo. Dolæ. *De furia podagra lacte victa & mitigata.* Amst 1707.

tended to all Sorts of vegetable Diet. In that Island are the first Physicians in all the World, according to the Judgment of Count *Lorenzo Magalotti*, a Man of the greatest Experience, Learning, and Honour: the Glory of being able to aspire to the second Place at least, he thought was reserved for his Countrymen, the *Tuscans*.

That the Gout may be prevented and cured, or very much mitigated by a Milk Diet, intermix'd with great Store of vegetable and very little of animal Food, we have more than one convincing Proof even in *Tuscany*. About seventeen Years ago, I proposed such a Method, in a Case I was consulted upon, and of which I then sent an Account over hither from *London* to a Friend, who dispersed many Copies of it: having then been also tried here by several gouty Persons. But not only the Gout and Pains of the Joints, may be taken away, or be remarkably alleviated by the *Pythagorean* Diet, but in general all the

Evils which arise from too great a Strength in the Solids, proceeding from the rancid, oily, and saline Acridity of the Fluids, from their too gross Consistency, from their heavy and tenacious Sediment, and from the too lively Activity of the internal moving Forces.

Thus Experience has shewn that we may cure by this Method the Rheumatism and Melancholy: two nervous and most troublesome Diseases, which reside chiefly in the Stomach and Intestines: as well as some other Disorders of the Nerves; likewise a Consumption, or Corruption of the Glands and Viscera, attended with a slow and habitual Fever, provided it is not gone beyond a certain Degree; also Aneurisms, if not extremely great, Obstructions, and the Scurvy. Of which Scurvy, tho' all do not take Notice of it from the first, there are many such Symptoms and Effects, as are observed in tedious and difficult Distempers; tho' they are called by other Names, and often mistaken, by many

of

of those ignorant Pretenders in Medicine, that sometimes get into their Hands the most worthy and best Sort of People. And of this Efficacy of the *Pythagorean* Diet, accommodated to the Circumstances of the Case, we have often seen Examples in this City beyond all common Expectation.

But what should fully perswade every one that thinks justly of the Salubrity and Power of vegetable Diet, is the Consideration of the horrid Effects of totally abstaining from such a Diet, unless it be for a very short Time: Accounts of which we meet with fully and faithfully recorded, in the most interesting and most authentic Narrations of human Affairs. Wars, Sieges of Places, long Encampments, distant Voyages, the Peopling of uncultivated and maritime Countries, remarkable Pestilences, and the Lives of illustrious Men, administer to any one who understands the Laws of Nature, irresistible Evidences of the bad and venomous Consequences of a Diet contrary to that of fresh Vegetables; that is, of Matters,

ters, which, tho' originally vegetable, are yet become hard, dry, and ftale: and of animal Subftances, whether they are hard or frefh without any Mixture of Herbage or of Fruits.

This and no other was the Caufe of the Plague at *Athens*, fo well defcribed by *Thucydides*, and I dare fay of the greateft Part alfo of the other Plagues, whereof we have faithful Accounts, as well as of many epidemical Diftempers, which may be obferved, to be almoft always accompanied with the Misfortune, either of a ftrait hoftile Siege, or a friendly Embargo by a miftaken Caution, or fome great Cold or Drynefs, which has deftroyed the Herbage, or render'd it by its Dearnefs or fome other Means not to be come at by the pooreft and loweft of the People: whence it is, that in fuch Circumftances, the Rich are wont to efcape the beft.

Thus we find that the Scurvy prevails as much where the Sun kills the Flowers and Plants, as where every green Thing is

cover'd

cover'd or destroy'd by the Ice or Snow; and that it is surprisingly cur'd by the short Use only of any fresh Vegetable, be it what it will; as also by a Decoction of the four Leaves cut from the first Tree we meet with. It is not a Northern Climate, not the Air of the Sea, nor the Salts of Flesh, but only an Abstinence from Vegetables which produces it. (1) Of this we have in every other Country, and in ours also very convincing Proofs; and we may observe the scorbutic Symptoms to prevail, more or less, in proportion to such Abstinence from Vegetables, whether through Necessity, or an unskilful Choice of Food; as is the Case at many Public Houses of Entertainment, where a common and ill-advised Frugality induces People to provide very dry Provisions, and such as can be kept a long time. And even in the Houses of some private Persons, who are rich, and tho' not ignorant, yet

---

(1) Bachstrom observation circa scorbutum Lupd Batav. 1734

yet are tenacious of Prejudices and learned Errors, we often meet with the true Scurvy, through such a voluntary Abstinence from Vegetables; owing to wrong Opinions in Medicine, which those are observed to be much the most exposed to, who believe there is not any thing in the Science of Physic.

Thus *Matthæus Curtius*, a famous Physician, to whom that magnificent Sepulchre in the *Campo santo di Pisa* was erected, is said to have shorten'd his Life, by eating nothing but Pidgeons, after he began to grow old, as *Cardan* (1) tells us of him. And we have known other Physicians no less esteem'd than *Curtius*, eminent Divines, and Lawyers, who, for want of this true and uncommon kind of Knowledge, have infected their Bodies with the Scurvy by a bad Regulation of their Diet; eating constantly strong Sauces, Eggs, forced Meats, and other Animal Food: without any Vegetables but only such as were dry'd

---

(1) De Sanitat tuenda. iii 16.

(73)

dry'd or preserv'd, without any Mixture of the more wholsome Sallads, or other fresh Herbs and Fruits.

Hereby we may also know the true Origin of the *Elephantiasis*, a Disease for which *Egypt* was infamous; and that in a much clearer manner than by supposing, as *Lucretius* (1) did, that it was occasion'd by the many morbid Semina floating in an unwholsome Air. The dreadful Symptoms of that Distemper, which *Aretæus* has represented in a lively manner, (2) with a kind of tragical Eloquence, and with singular physical Accuracy, will make those who have any Skill in that Art sensible, that the *Elephantiasis* of the Antients was no other than a high Degree of Scurvy; to which also those Ulcers of the Mouth may be reduc'd, which *Aretæus* (3) describes elsewhere, and which he tells us were call'd *Egyptiasis*, or *Siriasis*, be-

cause

(1) Lucret. vi. 11, 12.
(2) Aret. de signis & causis morbor. ii. 13.
(3) I. D.

cause frequent in those respective Counties.

When (1) *Galen* observ'd that such a Distemper was scarcely heard of in the more inland Countries of *Europe*, and especially among the Drinkers of Milk, but that it was frequent and dreadful among the common People of *Alexandria*, he reasoned thereupon like a worthy and skilful Physician as he was, and justly attributed the original Cause of it to their Diet: which, as he hints in many Places, and as other Authors agree, consisted of Meal, Pulse, dry Cheese, Fish, Scallops, Snakes, Ass's, and Camel's Flesh, and all other sorts of salt Provisions. To which if we add, that none but the rich People of that City, as *Aulus Issius* (2) tells us, had in their Houses Cisterns wherein the Water of the *Nile* clear'd itself down; but that the Multitude contented themselves with drinking it still thick and muddy; and that the Soil

of

---

(1) Ad Glaucon. li. 10.
(2) De bello Alexandr.

of that Country being naturally dry and saltish, should have laid them under a Necessity of bestowing much Water upon their sweet and tender Herbs, tho' with great Expence and Art, as (1) *Prosper Alpinus* relates, we shall easily be perswaded that the *Elephantiasis* was only an Effect of long Abstinence from fresh vegetable and wholsom Diet.

We may comprehend hereby, how rational the Remedy for this Distemper was that *Democritus* propos'd, of a Decoction of Herbs only, as *Aurelian* (2) asserts· or that prescrib'd by *Celsus*, (3) to abstain from all Food that was fat, glutinous and swelling; such being hard and difficult to be dissolved, and therefore of a Nature directly contrary to that of a fresh vegetable Diet; or that directed by *Aretæus*, (4) of the new gather'd Fruits of Trees, together

---

(1) De medic Ægypt p 16.
(2) Cel Aurel morb chronic. iv 1.
(3) Celf iii 25 cibis fine pinguibus, fine glutinosis, fine inflantibus
(4) Aret Curat. Diuturn. ii 13

ther with some Herbs and Roots, and abundance of Milk, either alone or mixt with Water; or, lastly, that Remedy of *Galen*'s, of Whey, and abundance of insipid Herbs: without regarding, in either of these Methods, any of the other fallacious and contrary Remedies, and particularly the so-much-boasted-of Flesh of Vipers, which has been for many Ages both a useless and dangerous Part of a Mountebank's Apparatus; Physic, even among the best of the Antients, abounding too much with mixt Medicines, many whereof were efficacious and good, but many others insignificant and bad; and which could not be distinguish'd from each other, with any reasonable Certainty, but by a more critical Knowledge of Nature, which is become much better understood in our Times, through the Improvement and united Assistance of various other Sciences.

We may conclude likewise from the scorbutic Nature of the *Elephantiasis*, that those

those Accounts may be true which are mention'd by the same *Aretæus*, (1) and which he did not dare to reject tho' they appear'd surprising and incredible; of some Persons afflicted with the *Elephantiasis*, who having (for Fear of the Contagion and the horrid Appearances of the Diseases upon them) been sent away from their Relations into the Mountains and Desarts, and there abandon'd, (as *Aurelius* affirms was then the common Custom) were afterwards found again alive and cur'd. But we should not believe that their Cure proceeded from their having eaten Vipers, as the Account relates, but rather from their total Abstinence from Animal Food, and a continual Use of Herbs, as more powerful philosophical Reasons induce us to believe.

It is hardly possible to conceive, how an Aversion to vegetable Food should ever have been propagated amongst Us in particular, since, if all Circumstances are rightly consider'd, it must appear that our City

(1) De causis & signis diuturn. ii 13.

City is one of the moſt healthy in the World; and principally for this Reaſon, that our common People are, from their Poverty, very little Eaters of Fleſh Meat: whereas, from the very Nature of our Soil, they are enabled, on the contrary, to procure, at the cheapeſt Rates, moſt Sorts of thoſe Herbs and Fruits, which are Delicacies ſcarcely ever ſo much as taſted in other Countries, but by thoſe of a much higher Rank. To which particular Conſtitution of our Country, that learned *Dutch* Phyſician *Adrianus Junius* ſeems to have alluded, who tranſlated the *Cæna Terreſtris* of *Plautus*, (1) " The *Florentine* " Herb Diet:" for otherwiſe ſuch an Expoſition would have been both falſe and ridiculous. It is then ſurely manifeſt, from the Reaſons above given, that when the Uſe of Vegetables has been long and plentiful, even tho' it be diſcontinu'd afterwards, it ſtill enables the Body to endure, without any bad Effects, the abſtaining

from

---

(1) Nomenc c xi. He died in 1575.

from them for a while, which People sometimes may find themselves constrained to by various Accidents of Life; and tho' many may, for the sake of gratifying their Palate, be still induc'd to give Animal Meats the Preference, sure we may at least conclude, that a Mixture of Vegetables with their Meat, would yet in some degree be serviceable, to mend the ill Qualities of their other Food.

But, notwithstanding vegetable Diet is not so displeasing to the Sense as may be commonly thought, Experience shews us, that any one who restrains himself, for a long time from Wine, and season'd Meats, will acquire a most exquisite Delicacy and distinguishing Sense of Tasting: the nervous Papillæ of the Tongue and Palate being less oppressed, and their Actions left more undisturbed, than by the redundant Quantity of the small pungent Particles with which Flesh, and spicy, hard, and oily Bodies so much abound: besides, in this Diet, altho' the Pleasure should really, in

some

some degree be diminished, in the mere Action of Eating, such is the Influence that Health has over all other Pleasures, and such the Efficacy of the *Pythagorean* Temperance, towards the procuring of Health and long Life, that those small Gratifications of the Senses, which are prevented by it, should be despised and hated by every ingenious Man, how voluptuous soever, that knows how little any real Pleasure can be tasted without a competent Share of Health. Nor were the Sentiments or Manners at all different of that great Philosopher of *Greece*, *Epicurus*, whose Doctrines were so much mistaken by the Vulgar, as to be looked upon as the Precepts of the most abandon'd Votary of Pleasure (1).

Others maintained, that vegetable Diet may too much diminish the Vigour and Strength of the Body, and, consequently, the Alacrity and Ability of the Mind; and, not to conceal any Thing, *Pythagoras* himself

---

(1) Laert x 11.

himself perswades a Champion, his Countryman, (1) to nourish himself with Flesh, whereby to acquire Strength superior to that of his Antagonists; and indeed the Experiment succeeded so well, that the Diet of the Wrestlers, which had before consisted of Cheese, dry'd Figs, Grain, Pulse, and other dry'd vegetable Matters, was from that Time quite alter'd. *Favorinus*, and *Laertius* himself have believed this of him; nor does it appear necessary to suppose another *Pythagoras* to have been the Author of this Advice, on account of our Philosopher's superstitious Opinion of the Transmigration of Souls, which it has been shewn that he did not really and literally believe. The famous *Milo* (2) of *Crotona*, who exceeded all Men in Strength of Body, and in being able to eat so large a Quantity of Meat, was also a Disciple, a Follower, and a Friend of *Pythagoras*,

---

(1) Laert. viii. 12. & 44.
(2) Athen. x. 1.

as *Strabo* (1) and other antient Writers affirm.

But the athletic Strength, resulting from an artificial Addition of Bulk to the Body, by a forc'd Diet (2) of many Flesh Meats, and other hard and oily sorts of Food, without fresh Vegetables or Water, together with Exercises contriv'd on Purpose, according to that Method, which, among the Antients, was reduc'd to a particular Art, was, in its own Nature, so far from being a healthy, robust, and vigorous Habit, that it was look'd upon as having a dangerous Tendency to many most grievous Diseases: whence procceded that wise and famous Advice of *Hippocrates*, for all such to subdue, as soon as possible, their over great Robustness, by Abstinence and medical Operations, who, not being Wrestlers by Profession, did nevertheless use that sort of Diet. *Plato* observes (3) that such People were

---

(1) Lib vi p 263 V. & Laert. viii 39, & Not Men g

(2) See the many antient Authors quoted by *Merc. Conr* 1 15 and by *Fab Agon* iii 1.

(3) De Republic lib iii p 404 & n 5.

were of a drowsy Disposition, and that, besides passing great Part of their Lives asleep, they were every now and then afflicted with some or other great and violent Distempers Galen (1) giving an Account more fully of the Disorders to which those Fools, he says, were usually subject, who, to give Pleasure to others by their Bravery, destroy'd their own Health, adds, that many of them, after a Combat, remain'd without Speech, Sense, or Motion, and were even seiz'd with a perfect Apoplexy, and suffocated by their own Bulk and Corpulency, or else by the bursting of some of their Blood-Vessels within them.

We find that such Accidents often happen to corpulent Persons, who feed much on high-season'd Flesh, and reject Herbs and Fruits, thereby losing that Equilibrium so necessary to be kept up, between the Fluids which move from the Heart to the extreme Parts, and those which return from those Parts to the Heart again: and for want

(1) De Republic. II. 18.

of which such Bodies fall easily into dropsical Disorders. Since therefore such fresh vegetable Food is compos'd, as *Celsus* observes, (1) of the tenderest Matters, and affords the least strong Nourishment, it should make up the greatest Portion of our Diet.

A genuine and constant Vigour of Body is the Effect of Health: which is much better preserv'd by an herbaceous, aqueous, sparing and tender Diet, than by one that is fleshy, vinous, unctious, hard, and in too great Abundance; and a healthy Body with a Mind clear, and accustom'd to suppress dangerous Inclinations, and to conquer unreasonable Passions, produces true Valour; which is the Reason, that among the Antients, some abstemious Nations, and such as liv'd wholly upon the Productions of the Earth, have been very great Warriors; and that this Frugality and Discipline of *Pythagoras* did not prevent any of his learned Followers from being very strong and couragious; as, amongst others, *Epimanondas*,

―――――――――――――――――――
(1) Ad Thrasyb cap 37.

Epimanondas, the *Theban*, so much prais'd for his civil and military Virtue, and for his *Pythagorean* Manner of Living and Thinking, was an Instance. (1) Many other eminent Captains, no less famous for their great Actions, than for their strict Temperance, are also recorded in the Histories of *Greece* and *Rome*.

The *Romans* were moreover so fully perswaded of the superior Goodness of vegetable Diet, that besides the private Examples of many of their great Men, they were willing to establish it by their Laws concerning Food, (2) amongst which were the *Lex Fannia* (3) and the *Lex Licinia*, which allowing but very little Flesh, permitted promiscuously, and without any Limitation, all manner of Things gather'd from the Earth, from Shrubs, and from Trees. And, agreeable to these Customs, we find the Sentiments of some, even of the *Roman* Emperors, to have been, altho'

---

(1) Diod except l vi Nep vita Epam Athen x 4.
(2) Gell. ii 24 Matrob. ii 13
(3) De Fannit Athen lib vi 21.

in other Things they thought themselves above all Regard to former Laws; we see that their most worthy Physicians and Philosophers were also of the same Opinion. *Antonius Musa*, who merited a publick Statue in *Rome* (1) for the perfect and happy Cure perform'd by him upon *Augustus*, made Use of *Lettice* (2) principally therein: and by his Advice it was that this great Prince came into that sparing and simple *Pythagorean* Diet, which *Suetonius* (3) minutely describes, consisting principally of Bread sopp'd in cold Water, and of some Sorts of Apples of an agreeable and vinous Acidity. *Horace* also made great Use of the *Pythagorean* Diet, as he tells us in many Places of his judicious and most excellent Poems, therein following, as we suppose, the Advice of the same *Musa*, who was his Physician.

We find the same Preference given to vegetable Food by all the other ancient

Latin

---

(1) Suet. Aug. 59.
(2) Plin. xix. 8. Divus certe Augustus lactuca con‍‍valitus in ægritudine prudentia Musæ medici fertur.
(3) Cap. 76 & 77.

Latin Writers, who had any Understanding of the Nature of Things, and by *Galen*, and *Plutarch*, who has shewed more particularly, perhaps than any one, the Danger of animal Diet, in his Precepts of Health, and in his Discourses on eating Flesh.

Nor has our Age been destitute of Examples of Men, brave from the Vigour both of their Bodies and Minds, who at the same time have been Drinkers of Water, and Eaters of Fruits and Herbs. In certain Mountains of *Europe*, there are People, even at this Time, who live on Herbs only and Milk; yet are very invincible and stout; and the *Japanese* (who are very resolute in despising Dangers, and even Death itself) abstain from all animal Food; and there are besides a thousand Examples known to every one, of Nations and Persons of great Temperance, joined with all other consummate Virtues.

The vulgar Opinion, which condemns Vegetables, and so highly cries up the

Use of animal Food as conducive to Health, being therefore so ill grounded, I always judg'd it proper to oppose it; moved thereto both by my Experience, and that little Knowledge of natural Things, which some Study, and the Conversation of great Men has led me into. And now thinking, that this my constant Perseverance may have been honoured by some learned and prudent Physicians in their own Practice, which cannot but have great Authority with others; I have thought it my Duty thus publickly to set forth the Reasons for the *Pythagorean* Diet, considered as fit to be used in Medicine, and at the same time perfectly innocent, well adapted to Temperance, and greatly beneficial and conducive to Health. It is also by no Means destitute of a certain delicate Voluptuousness, of a gentile and even splendid Luxury, if we employ Curiosity and Art, in the Choice and Abundance of the best fresh vegetable Aliments, which the Fertility

tility and natural Difpofition of our own fine Country feems, as it were, to invite us to. And fo much the more was I induced to treat on this Argument, from the Hopes I have, that it may, perhaps, entertain the Reader by its Novelty; there not being, that I know of, any Book purpofely wrote on this Subject, and which endeavours to point out, exactly, the Original and the Reafons of it.

I have been defirous to prove, by fuch Means as the two Arts Criticifm and Medicine have furnifh'd me with, that *Pythagoras*, the firft Inventor of the frefh vegetable Diet, was both a very great Philofopher and an able Phyfician, and no Stranger to the moft cultivated and difcreet good Breeding, a prudent and experienc'd Man, whofe Motive for the fo much commending and introducing his Way of Life, was not any Superftition or Extravagance, but a Defire to be affifting to the Health and good Behaviour of Mankind, for which

Reason he made no Scruple of intermixing it, occasionally, sometimes even with animal Food: that such *Pythagorean* Diet, consider'd as a Remedy, is perfectly agreeable to all that can be requir'd in the most exact Knowledge of modern Physick; and that it is very powerful to prevent, remove, or mitigate many of the most violent, and obstinate Maladies to which we are subject, as both Reason and Experience perswade us, since, of late Years, it has again been introduc'd into the most noble and safest Practice of Physic.

From all which it appears, how well those among us would deserve, for promoting the Health of Mankind, to whom Fortune has given Estates, and bestowed her choicest Gifts, in the magnificent Seats that so beautifully adorn the Plains and the Hills of our native *Tuscany*; if, after the Example of some of the greatest of

the

the *Romans*, they would place Part of their Glory in introducing among us new Fruits and Herbage, and in a more diligent Culture of their delicious Gardens; from whence the rest of the People also might enjoy the valuable Effects of their learned Opulency.

F I N I S.

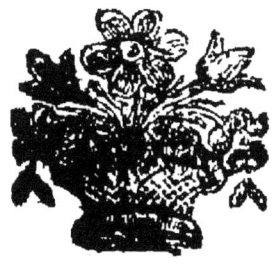

Lightning Source UK Ltd.
Milton Keynes UK
UKHW052346161121
394065UK00019B/912